Pharmacological Considerations Of Certain Diseases And   Anesthesia

HALA MOSTAFA GOMA

Professor of Anesthesia Cairo University

Table of contents

Introduction

Patient undergoing surgical operation under anesthesia ,may be has a concomitant diseases .the chronic administration of this drug may be interact with anesthetics by many route.it may be affect patients systems which is in turn may lead to modification of anesthetic technique ,or interact with anesthetic drugs leads to avoid certain anesthetics, or reduction of the dose needed.

The anesthesia must be aware with these drugs ,about their side effects, full preoperative history is needed, proper evaluation of the systems affected ,for example chemotherapy drugs have a cardiac toxicity ,pulmonary toxicity ,hepatorenal,and coagulation abnormalities .immuno supressents for auto immune diseases ,mythenia gravis ,and others can affect plan of anesthesia .

This book focused on some of common diseases facing anesthetist and be a challenge to produce safe anesthesia.

Cardiac diseases

Rheumatic heart diseases

1. Antibiotics prophylaxis against infected endocarditis

- For a long time cardiologists have routinely recommended antibiotic prophylaxis (ABP) at the time of dental procedures in patients deemed to be at risk of infective endocarditis (IE).
- The BSAC guidelines recommended withdrawal of ABP for the majority of patients limiting them to individuals perceived to be at the highest risk of IE (e.g. a prior history of IE, prosthetic cardiac valves and surgically constructed pulmonary or system shunts/conduits). These guidelines were welcomed by the majority of dentists and microbiologists as a step in the right direction.

2. Prophylaxis against embolization:

Anticoagulant therapy is administered to prolong the prothrombin time to 1.5 to 2.0 times control, using rabbit brain thromboplastin (standardized international normalized ratio = 3.0 to 4.5).

Because intracardiac thrombus formation may start during and continues early after operation, restarting heparin therapy 6 hours after operation and continuing it for the duration of the hospitalization is advised. For mechanical prosthetic heart valves, oral anticoagulation as outlined plus dipyridamole is advised indefinitely. Platelet inhibitor therapy alone is insufficient.

1. <u>Ischemic heart diseases</u>

ß-adrenoceptor blockade (e.g., propranolol (Inderal); metoprolol (Lopressor)

- Reduces cardiac O_2 demand by attenuating contractility (negative inotropism) increases mediated by increased circulating catecholamines levels and sympathetic nervous system activity
- Reduced heart rate (negative chronotropism) increases diastolic filling time, thereby increasing time available for coronary vascular perfusion
- It reduced myocardial oxygen consumption (reduced afterload)
- reduced coronary blood flow through stenotic regions
- both limitation in myocardial oxygen demand and maximization of supply: anesthetic should optimize this balance

Monitor ventricular filling pressures using the pulmonary artery catheter

Nitroglycerin may be used to maintain optimal filling pressure

4. Optimization of coronary perfusion pressure gradients involved typically:

- Raising the diastolic arterial pressure
- Decreasing LVEDP (left ventricular and diastolic pressure)
- With left ventricular heart failure, inotropic support may improve the relationship between oxygen supply and demand
- autoimmunity is known to have a genetic basis and tends to cluster in families as different autoimmune diseases
- Different ethnic groups are more susceptible to certain autoimmune diseases.

Autoimmune diseases

- Women respond to infection, vaccination, and trauma with increased antibody production, whereas inflammation is usually more severe in men resulting in an increased mortality in men and protection against infection in women
- Women respond to infection, vaccination, and trauma with increased antibody production, whereas inflammation is usually more severe in men resulting in an increased mortality in men and protection against infection in women

.

Anesthetic drug and immunosuppressive drugs

Azathioprine, an antimetabolite immunosuppressor, may interact with muscle relaxants, and dose increases of 37% with cisatracurium, 20% with vecuronium, and 45% with pancuronium

Patients on corticosteroid therapy should continue therapy and may require stress dosing

General anesthesia and MS

- Immuno-suppresion occurs with the use of all the alkylating agents. Meticulous attention must be given to aseptic techniques in the perioperative period in order to avoid potentially lethal iatrogenic infection.
- General anesthesia is most often used in patients with multiple sclerosis.
- Succinylcholine judiciously as demyelination and denervation may increase the risk of succinylcholine-induced hyperkalemia in these patients.
- Nondepolarizing neuromuscular blockers are safe to use although patients with multiple sclerosis may have altered sensitivity to these drugs in the setting of baseline limb weakness.
- They may also have limited 'physiologic reserve' (neurologic and respiratory) and be less able to tolerate stressors such as a mild degree of post-operative residual muscle relaxant.
- As in other patients with chronic brain injury, patients with MS may be expected to have some MAC reduction and delayed emergence proportionate to the severity of their disease.

Myasthenia Gravis

Myasthenia Gravis is an autoimmune disease that attacks post-synaptic nicotinic acetylcholine receptors at the NMJ.

- There is muscle weakness and fatigue
- Ocular, bulbar (muscles involved in speech, chewing and swallowing), respiratory, and proximal skeletal muscles.
- Symptoms seem to be worse at the end of the day or after exertion.
- These patients can pose a challenge during anesthesia not only because of their disease process but also from the medications used to treat them (acetylcholinesterase inhibitors, steroids, etc.).
- These patients can pose a challenge during anesthesia not only because of their disease process but also from the medications used to treat them (acetylcholinesterase inhibitors, steroids, etc.).
- Patients with MG are resistant to succinylcholine and are exquisitely sensitive to non-depolarizing NMBs.
- Patients with involvement of respiratory or bulbar muscles tend to have a higher risk for aspiration
- Pretreatment with metoclopramide or H2 blockers may be helpful.

- Some patients are sensitive to respiratory depressants and premedication with opioids, BZDs, or barbiturates should be considered carefully or not at all.

Idiopathic thrombocytopenic purpura (ITP)

- Severe thrombocytopenia in ITP requires platelet transfusion before surgery.
- IV immunoglobulin 1 g/kg reduce platelet destruction
- Perioperative methylprednisolone 1 g along with pre-operative 8 RDP transfusions covered the perioperative period.
- Each unit of RDP is assumed to increase the platelet count by 3000–5000 units/mm 3.

Thromboelastography can help us in this scenario, but it was not available with us. Tranexamic acid, an antifibrinolytic, helps to reduce operative blood loss and blood transfuse

- Non-steroidal anti-inflammatory drugs (NSAIDs) including paracetamol were avoided.

No intramuscular injections were given.
- Commonly used disease-modifying drugs (DMDs) include methotrexate, hydroxychloroquine, sulfasalazine, infliximab (Remicade), etanercept (Enbrel), and leflunomide (Arava, inhibits dihydroorotate dehydrogenase which is involved in

pyrimidine synthesis).Patients may also be on NSAIDs and/or glucocorticoids

Hypothyroidism

Hypothyroid patients require less preoperative sedation and are prone to drug-induced respiratory depression,

- benadryl for sedation,
- metoclopramide for gastric-emptying (which is slowed).
- Euthyroid patients may receive their usual dose of thyroid medication on the morning of surgery .

Cardiac complications

- diminished cardiac output,
- Blunted baroreceptor reflexes, and decreased intravascular volume, are at risk for severe hypotension.
- Induction may be best accomplished with ketamine
- . Consider pancuronium as a paralytic agent (chronotropic effects).
- Do NOT give volatile anesthetics to hypothyroid patients, as they are at risk for severe myocardial depression.
- Consider nitrous oxide plus intravenous agents (ex. benzodiazepines).
- There is no evidence that hypothyroid patients have reduced MAC requirements.

Causes of delayed recovery from general anesthesia

- hypothermia,
- respiratory depression,
- slowed drug biotransformation
- hypothyroid patients often require prolonged mechanical ventilation
- opiates may need to be avoided to avoid respiratory depression

- Ketorolac for postoperative analgesia

Pheochromocytoma:

- pre-established alpha-blockade (ex. phenoxybenzamine, prazosin)
- Treat any arrhythmias if present (beta blockers).

- Note that alpha-blockers will enhance insulin release, decreasing blood glucose levels
- Fentanyl and IV lidocaine should be considered prior to intubation.

- Pancuronium should be avoided (because of its SNS stimulating effects). Nitroprusside should be available at induction.
- Volatiles, which are ideal as they blunt the SNS.
- If MAC 1.5-2.0 does not adequately control blood pressure,
- nitroprusside infusion should probably be started.

- Note that when the veins are ligated, circulating catecholamines will drop rapidly, necessitating a reduction in volatile anesthesia as well as fluid resuscitation. Hyperglycemia (due to reduced alpha-induced insulin production) may ensue, thus glucose should be checked with regularity.
- Droperidol should be avoided, as it has been shown to cause a paradoxical hypertensive response (thought to be due to inhibition of norepinephrine reupdate.

Anesthetic Dose requirement for obese patient
- Water soluble drugs as muscle relaxant adjusted according to lean body weight
- Fat soluble drugs as volatile anesthesia and narcotics Rarely need to dose based on more than 80 kg for females or 100 kg for males
- [Many drugs accumulate in adipose tissue, further complicating management, although obese patients may not be at increased risk for delayed emergenc.
- Obese patients have larger volumes of distribution for opiates and benzodiazepines (fat-soluble), thus some authors recommend larger loading doses and lower/less-frequent maintenance doses.
- Obese patients usually require 20–25% less local anesthetic (epidural fat, distended veins) and are at particular risk for respiratory compromise.
-

- deep venous thrombosis, and pulmonary embolism heparin should be considerd.

Diabetes

- Patients e on ACE-inhibitors (because of their renal sparing effects) or ARBs and may be at risk for severe hypotension at induction.
- Bradycardia non-responsive to atropine has been described in diabetic surgery patients
- DKA should be treated with fluid resuscitation, IV insulin (0.2 U/kg initially, 0.1 U/kg/hr after, goal is to decrease by 75–100 mg/dL or 10% per hour), and K+ supplementation (some, but not all, authors recommend bicarbonate if pH is 7.2).
- Oral hypoglycemic doses are often held the morning of surgery, as patients are NPO and the risk of hypoglycemia is real.
- Metformin and sulfonylureas are often held for 24-48 hours before surgery. Metformin also carries with it the risk of metabolic acidosis.

- Insulin-dependent diabetics should receive insulin preoperatively, although there is no standardized dose – most commonly, ½ the daily dose is given as an intermediate acting agent after an IV is placed and glucose is checked

Intraoperative Management

- IV lidocaine may help facilitate glycemic control [
- Insulin-dependent diabetics should have glucose monitored every 1-2 hours, with a goal of keeping glucose < 180.
- Do not rely on SQ or IM insulin intraoperatively, as these routes rely on adequate tissue perfusion.
- Consider starting a dedicated IV for D5W and IV insulin infusions (which could potentially interfere with other medications).

Cancer

Epidural anesthesia

- Opiate-enhanced epidural is used, consider a lipophilic drug (ex.fentanyl),
- Morphine will potentially spread rostrally,
- Potentially causing mental status changes and respiratory depression.
- Consider 0.5% bupivacaine intraoperatively, followed by 0.125% – 0.25% post-operatively.
- In patients for whom an epidural is not possible, consider ketamine at 0.2 mg/kg/hr after a 0.5 mg/kg bolus, as well as gabapentin 600-1200 mg PO.

System toxicity	Chemotherapeutic agents
Cardiac toxicity	Busulphan, cisplatin, cyclophosphamide, daunorubucin, 5-fluorouracil
Pulmonarytoxicity	Methotrexate, bleomycin, busulphan, cyclophosphamide, cytarabine, carmustine
Renal toxicity	Methotrexate, L-asparginase, carboplatin, ifosfamide, mitomycin-C
Hepatic toxicity	Actinomycin D, methotrexate, androgens, L-asparginase, busulphan, cisplatinum, azathioprine
CNS toxicity	Methotrexate, cisplatin, interferon, hydroxyurea, procarbazine, vincristine
SIADH secretion	Cyclophosphamide, vincristine

Cardiovascular effects and complications following chemotherapy
Anthracyclines; i.e. doxorubicin (adriamycin), daunorubicin, and epirubicinare the commonest agents implicated in the development of cardiac toxicity after cancer chemotherapy.

Three types depending on their appearance in relation to timing of therapy,

Anthracycline agents may impair myocardial contractility.

Risk factors for development of anthracycline cardiotoxicity:

1. high dose radiation to the mediastinum
2. concurrent cyclophosphamide therapy
3. extremes of age,
4. prior ischemic heart disease,
5. hypertension,
6. valvular heart disease and liver diseases.
7. Cumulative dose in the range of 300-450 mg/m2 is about 1-10%, while doses higher than this invites a risk of>30%.

Pathogenesis ofanthracycline cardiotoxicity:

- The anthracycline antibiotics react with cytochrome P-450 reductase in the presence of reduced nicotinamide adenine dinucleotide phosphateto form semiquinone radical intermediates, which in turn can react with oxygen to form superoxide anion radicals.

These can generate both hydrogen peroxide and hydroxylradicals, which are highly destructive to cells thus causing myofibrillarlysis, cytoplasmic vacuolization, and degeneration of nuclei and mitochondria in the myocytes.

- diffuse uptake on imaging indicates a generalised process such as anthracycline cardiomyopathy; a focal uptake will suggest local pathology such as myocardial infarct.mitoxantrone at a total dose of more than 140 mg/m2 can suffer congestive heart failure
- anthracycline-induced cardiomyopathy.

Dysrhythmias:

- dysrhythmias unrelated to the cumulative dose
- Dysrhythmias may occur hours or even days after administration.
- Commonly observed dysrhythmias include supraventricular tachycardia, complete heart blocks, and ventricular tachycardia.
- Doxorubicin may prolong the QT interval.
- anthracyclines may enhance the myocardial depressive effect of anesthetics even in patients with normal resting cardiac function.
- cyclophosphamide causes myocardial tissue injury
- A cyclophosphamide dose range of more than 120mg.kg−1 over 2 days can result in severe congestive heart failure and haemorrhagic myocarditis, pericarditis, and necrosis.
- busulfan oral daily dosage may suffer endocardial fibrosis, with signs and symptoms of constrictive cardiomyopathy.
- Patients with preexisting cardiac disease receiving interferon in conventional doses may have exacerbations of their underlying illness.
- mitomycin for extended periods of time and dosages has been shown to produce myocardial damage.

- <u>paclitaxel,</u> with cisplatinum, may also produce ventricular tachycardia
-

Acute and Subacute cardiotoxicity:
- It can occur immediately after a single dose or a course of anthracycline therapy.
- Acute toxicity commonly (40%) takes the form of ECG changes such as nonspecific ST-T changes, decreased QRS voltage, and QT prolongation
- Decreased R wave amplitude has been thought by some to signal development of chronic cardiomyopathy later, though it is not proved.
- Sinus tachycardiais the most common rhythm disturbance but avariety of arrhythmias, including ventricular, supraventricular, and junctional tachycardia, have been reported.
- Atrioventricular and bundle-branch block have.
- These changes occur at all dose intervals and except for decreased QRS voltage, resolve 1 to 2 months after cessation of the therapy.
- Sudden death may also occur, due to ventricular fibrillation.
- Rare cases of subacute cardiotoxicity resulting in acute failure of the left ventricle, pericarditis or a fatal pericarditis-myocarditis syndrome, particularly in children, have been reported.

- If these patients recover they should not receive further treatment with anthracyclines.
- In elderly patients with preexisting heart disease, congestive heart failure can occur, which is generally transient and responds to normal medical management.

Chronic or late cardiotoxicity:

- Chronic cardiotoxicity after anthracyclines classically takes the form of cardiomyopathy. CXR review may reveal cardiomegaly.
- ECG changes occur with these agents and includenon-specific ST-and T-wave changes, prematureatrial and ventricular contractions, sinus tachycardia and low-voltage QRS complexes.
- Anthracycline cardiotoxicity is a cumulative dose related phenomenon.
- The incidence of congestive heart failure secondary to anthracycline induced cardiotoxicity increases with dose.
- The rapid increasein incidence of CHF after a dose of 550 mg/m2 has made it a popular empiric-limiting dose for doxorubicin-induced cardiotoxicity.

Late onset cardiotoxicity:

- occultventricular dysfunction, heart failure and arrhythmias occurring in previously asymptomatic patients more than a year after anthracycline therapy.

- Doxorubicin can cause subclinical myocardial injury during pre-adolescent years and this in later years retards appropriate growth of the myocardium during growth spurt.

- Anthracycline treated patients under anaesthesia can develop acute intraoperative left ventricular failure refractory to β-adrenergic receptor agonists.
- Amrinone and sulmazole are the new class of cardiotonics with inotropic drugs useful in such conditions.

Pulmonary effects and complications of cancer chemotherapy
- 75% to 90% of pulmonary complications are secondary to infection.
- The cancer patient can suffer infectious complications secondary to chemotherapy (e.g., Bleomycin), thoracic radiation, and multiple pulmonary resections.
- respiratory failure in cancer patients requiring assisted mechanical ventilation is associated with a 75% mortality rate
- Pulmonary infiltrates seen on a routine chest radiograph is extensive; there are many causes for such infiltrates.
- busulfan, cyclophosphamide, paclitaxel, etc, can lead to pulmonary complications. Bleomycin, an antitumour agent, producing lung damage.

bleomycin pulmonary toxicity produced by have been described:

- About 0-40% patients are reportedto develop pulmonary toxicity

- 11-30% patients will have non-lethal pulmonary fibrosis and the mortality associated with bleomycin toxicity will range from 2-10%.

- Another mechanism for bleomycin toxicity involves the production of superoxide and other free radical moieties, Cleave nuclear DNA.

- The production of these highly oxidizing radicals might be increased by the inspiration of fortified concentrations of oxygen.

Pathology of chemotherapy pulmonary toxicity

- Dose dependent interstitial pneumonitis progressing to chronic fibrosis

- An acute hypersensitivity pneumonitis with peripheral eraleosinophilia resembling eosinophilic pneumonia.

- An acute chest pain syndrome.

- A bronchitis obliterans with organising pneumonia.

- Pulmonary veno-occlusive disease.

- Progressive interstitial pneumonitis and fibrosis is the most common pattern of bleomycin lung injury.

Renal complications:-

- Cisplatinum, a commonly used anticancer drug has been found to produce toxic effects like nephrotoxicity, myelosuppression, neuropathy in stocking and glove distribution, auditory and visual impairment.

- The dose-limiting factor for single agent use, however, is nephrotoxicity. 30% of patients receiving cisplatinum will develop nephrotoxicity, especially if the hydration is not properly controlled.

Mechanism of renal complications of chemothrapy

- It causes coagulation necrosis of proximal and distal renal tubular epithelial cells and in the collecting ducts leading to are duction in the renal blood flow and glomerular filtration rate (GFR).

- Cisplatinum leads to wasting of magnesium and potassium. A single dose of 2mg/kg or 50-75mg/m2 will produce nephrotoxicity in 25-30% of patients.

- The newer analogues of cisplatinum, such as carboplatinum and oxaloplatinum are less nephrotoxic with equal efficacy in controlling the malignancy.

- Methotrexate causes the acute nephrotoxicity as a result of its intratubular precipitation

Acute renal failure

- Acute renal failure can result within 24 hours of administration of a single dose of cisplatinum.
- Use of normal saline is particularly beneficial as high chloride concentrations in the tubules inhibit the hydrolysis of cisplatinum.
- The renal toxicity may be accentuated if the patient receives aminoglycosides concomitantly
-

CNS complications:-

- Vinca alkaloids were the first anticancer drugs found to have neurotoxiceffects.
- Vincristine is probably the only drug whose dose limiting toxicityis neurotoxicity.
- It can affect the central, peripheral or the autonomic nervous systems. Peripheral neuropathies present as peripheral paresthesias with depression of deep tendon reflexes.
- The paresthesias progress proximally with therapy. Motor dysfunction and gait disorders can occur.
- Vincristine, vinblastine, procarbazine, cisplatinum
- all can cause a toxic neuropathy with paresthesia, loss of deep tendon reflexes and muscle weakness.

- Autonomic neuropathy with orthostatic hypotension is a rare concomitant of neoplasia
- Cranial nerve effects may manifest as opthalmoplegia and facial palsy
- Autonomic neuropathy can present asorthostatic hypotension, erectile dysfunction, constipation, difficulty in micturition, bladder atony, et
- Cisplatinum, along with its effects on the kidney also affects the nervous system. 50% patients receiving cisplatinum will display neurotoxicity depending on dose and treatment duration. It generally takes the form of paresthesias.
- Continued treatment will lead to loss of deep tendon reflexes, vibration sense and sensory ataxia.

Hepatic complications:-
- Hepatocellular dysfunction is manifested as raised serum enzymes,
- fatty infiltration of liver and cholestasis, due to direct toxic effect of the drug or it's metabolite.
- L-asparginase and cytarabine are most commonly implicated agents in hepatocellular dysfunction.
- A decreased synthetic function with low proteins and coagulation abnormalities may be seen.Ascites, painful hepatomegaly, and encephalopathy may result after administration of cytarabine, cyclophosphamide, mitomycin, etc.

- Bone marrow function in cancer patients may be disturbed by primary bone marrow disorders (e.g., leukemia), bony metastases (e.g., from breast cancer), as well as myelosuppressive chemotherapy.
- The production of any or all blood elements may be impaired. There is dysfunctional coagulation. The PT and PTT are shortened. There is increase in factor I, V, VIII, IX, XI and FDP.
- There is reduced survival of the platelets and the decreased antithrombin III activity.
- Some investigators have maintained a minimal level

Syndrome of inappropriate antidiuretic hormone secretion (SIADH):-

- Another metabolic abnormality in patients with cancer like lung, pancreas-adeno-carcinoma, duodenum, thymoma, mesothelioma, leukaemia, hodgkin, reticulum cell sarcoma, is SIADH, which occurs in 1% to2% of cancer patients.
- Some drugs, such as vasopressin, carbamazepine, oxytocin, vincristine, vinblastine, cyclophosphamide, phenothizianes, tricyclic antidepressant agents, narcotics, and monoamine oxidase inhibitors, can also induce SIADH.

Steroid administration:

- The oncology patient often has a history of exogenous glucocorticoid administration a as part of a chemotherapy regimen.
- The physician at the time of pre-operative evaluation has to decide on the use and the amount of stress steroid coverage.
- The patient who has received ≥2 weeks of glucocorticoids within the past year is considered at risk for adrenal suppression.
- However, many of these patients are capable of a normal stress response. The corticotrophin (ACTH) stimulation test is the definitive test to identify adrenal suppression.

Tumorlysis syndrome:-
- Chemotherapy induces rapid tumor cell lysis in patients with a large malignant cell burden over an exquisitely sensitive tumor
- This classically occurs in patients with Burkitt's lymphoma, non-Hodgkin's lymphomas, acute lymphoblastic and nonlymphoblastic leukemias, and chronic myelogenous leukemia.

- In addition, it may also occur continuously in patients with lymphomas and leukemia following treatment with chemotherapy, radiation, glucocorticoids, tamoxifen, or interferon. The clinical mani-festations of this syndrome are related to the metabolic abnormalities.

- In those patients with suspected tumor lysis syndrome or for those patients who receive chemotherapeutic agents likely to induce the syndrome, prevention is the mainstay of treatment.
- To prevent the development of acute renal failure, patients who are to undergo treatment for malignancies should receive vigorous intravenous hydration, often with diuretics or renal doses of dopamine to ensure adequate urine output

Chemotherapy and wound healing:-
- The outcome of surgical procedures may be affected by the wound-healing impairment caused by antineoplastic agents used to treat the underlying tumor. The neutropenia that accompanies some chemotherapy within 7 to 10 days of administration can interfere with the early phases of wound healing..
- The effects of chemotherapy directly on wound healing depend on doseand the timing of drug administration relative to creation of the wound.
- A high incidence of wound complications has been reported in women undergoing mastectomy after receiving preoperative chemotherapy and radiation. Bleomycin has not been associated with increased wound complications.

Drugs cause osteoporosis

1. Steroid-induced osteoporosis (SIOP) arises due to use of glucocorticoids – analogous to Cushing's syndrome and involving mainly the axial skeleton. The synthetic glucocorticoid prescription drug prednisone is a main candidate after prolonged intake. Some professional guidelines recommend prophylaxis in patients who take the equivalent of more than 30 mg hydrocortisone (7.5 mg of prednisolone), especially when this is in excess of three months. Alternate day use may not prevent this complication.

2. Barbiturates, phenytoin and some other enzyme-inducing antiepileptic – these probably accelerate the metabolism of vitamin D.

3. L-Thyroxin over-replacement may contribute to osteoporosis, in a similar fashion as thyrotoxicosis does. This can be relevant in subclinical hypothyroidism.

4. drugs induce hypogonadism, for example aromatase inhibitors used in breast cancer, methotrexate and other

antimetabolite drugs, depot progesterone andgonadotropin-releasing hormone agonists.

5. Anticoagulants – long-term use of heparin is associated with a decrease in bone density, and warfarin (and related coumarins) have been linked with an increased risk in osteoporotic fracture in long-term use.

6. Proton pump inhibitors – these drugs inhibit the production of stomach acid; this is thought to interfere with calcium absorption. Chronic phosphate binding may also occur with aluminum-containing antacids.

7. Thiazolidinediones (used for diabetes) – rosiglitazone and possibly pioglitazone, inhibitors of PPARγ, have been linked with an increased risk of osteoporosis and fracture.

8. Chronic lithium therapy has been associated with osteoporosis.

selective serotonin reuptake inhibitors (SSRIs)

- Drugs in this group include amitriptyline, imipramine, desipramine, doxepin, nortriptyline and others.
- Desipramine and nortriptyline are used as tricyclic antidepressant as they are less-sedating.

TCAs

- inhibit synaptic reuptake of norepinephrine and serotonin.
- they also affect other neurochemical systems including histaminergic and cholinergic systems.

Side-effects

- Postural hypotension
- Cardiac dysrhythmias
- Urinary retention
- Dry mouth
- Blurred vision and sedation.

ECG

- T wave changes, widening of the QRS complex and prolongation of QT interval, bundle branch block or other conduction abnormalities, or PVCs.
- Ventricular arrhythmias and refractory hypotension may occur at higher doses.

Anesthesia and TCA

Increase anesthetic requirements, increased availability of neurotransmitters in the central nervous system .

anticholinergics

- Atropine cross the blood–brain barriermay cause postoperative confusion.
- Exaggerated blood pressure responses following administration of indirect acting
- Vasopressors such as ephedrine due to increased availability of norepinephrine at the post-synaptic nervous

 Pancuronium, ketamine, meperidine and epinephrine containing solutions should be avoided.

Depression:
1. Exaggerated response to both indirect acting vasopressors
2. Sympathetic stimulation
3. If hypotension occurs and vasopressors are needed, direct acting drugs such as phenylephrine are recommended. The dose should probably be decreased to minimize the likelihood of an exaggerated hypertensive response.
4. During anesthesia and surgery, it is important to avoid stimulating the sympathetic nervous system.

Potentiating the cardiac depressant effects of anesthetic agents

Chronic therapy with tricyclic antidepressant drugs depletes cardiac catecholamine.

Selective serotonin reuptake inhibitors (SSRIs

Mechanism of action:
- SSRIs block reuptake of serotonin at the pre-synaptic membranes,
- With relatively little effect on adrenergic, cholinergic, histaminergic or other neurochemical systems.

Side-effects
- They are associated with few side-effects.
- Examples include fluoxetine, paroxetine and sertraline.
- Headache, agitation and insomnia.

- Among SSRIs, fluoxetine is a potent inhibitor of certain hepatic cytochrome P-450 enzymes.
- This drug may increase the plasma concentration of drugs that depend upon hepatic metabolism for clearance, such as warfarin, theophylline, phenytoin and benzodiazepines.
- Antidysarrhythmic drugs are also metabolized by this enzyme system, and fluoxetine inhibition of the enzyme system may result in potentiation of their effects.

Anesthetic precaution with SSRIs

SSRIs should be continued throughout the perioperative period to prevent discontinuation syndrome.

Avoid the use of pethidine, tramadol, pentazocine and dextromethorphan.

Serotonin syndrome

Serotonin syndrome is a potentially life-threatening adverse drug reaction that results from increased serotonin levels in the brain stem and spinal cord. A large number of drugs have been associated with the serotonin syndrome.

These include SSRI, MAOI, TCAs, pethidine, tramadol and dextromethorphan.

Clinical features

- Behaviour (agitation and confusion),
- Increased motor activity and autonomic instability (hyperthermia, tachycardia, labile blood pressure and diarrhea.

- Seizures, rhabdomyolysis, renal failure, arrhythmias, coma and death may

MAOIs

MAOIs, tranylcypromine and phenelzine, and the selective and reversible MAOIs, moclobemide,

MECHANISM OF ACTION

MAOIs

MAOIs, tranylcypromine and phenelzine, and the selective and reversible MAOIs, moclobemide,

MECHANISM OF ACTION

- Inhibition of the metabolic breakdown of norepinephrine and serotonin by the MAO enzyme.
- The level of norepinephrine and serotonin is increased at the receptor site. All MAOIs are eliminated by hepatic metabolism

Interactions between MAOIs and anaesthetic drugs

There are two distinct types of reaction that can occur between MAOIs and opioids.

CLINICAL PICTURE

Serotonin syndrome

- pethidine and dextromethorphan remain contraindicated.
- Other opioids like morphine, fentanyl, alfentanyl and remifentanyl can all be used safely.

Type II (depressive) reaction

- It is very rare, is thought to be due to MAO inhibition of hepatic enzymes resulting in enhanced effects of all opioids.
- It is reversed by naloxone.

Indirect acting sympathomimetics

- It precipitates potentially fatal hypertensive crisis and are absolutely contraindicated with any MAOIs.
- Direct acting sympathomimetics (adrenaline, noradrenaline and phenylephrine) may have an enhanced effect due to receptor hypersensitivity
- Dosages should be titrated.
- Phenelzine decreases plasma cholinesterase concentration and prolongs the action of suxamethonium.
- Pancuronium should be avoided as it releases stored noradrenaline.
- MAOIs may cause a reduction in the hepatic metabolism of barbiturates, resulting in reduction of the dose requirement of thiopentone.
- Propofol and etomidate can be used safely. Ketamine should be avoided as it causes sympathetic stimulation.
- Local anesthetics containing adrenaline should be used with caution.

- Benzodiazepines, inhalational anesthetic agents, anticholinergic drugs and non-steroidal anti-inflammatory drugs can be used safely in patients taking MAOIs.

Anesthesia for a patient on MAOIs

- MAOI is to be stopped, the doses should be reduced gradually and with regular psychiatric review.
- Cancellation of surgery should be avoided and the treatment restarted as soon as possible post-operatively.
- In a patient on MAOIs or in the emergency situation, benzodiazepine premedication can be given and sympathetic stimulation should be avoided. Adequate hydration of the patient should be ensured.
- Hypotension should be treated initially with intravenous fluids and then with cautious doses of phenylephrine.
- Pethidine and indirect acting sympathomimetics are absolutely contraindicated

- The interactions between antipsychotics and anesthetic patients with hysteria require less anesthetic agents than those with neurotic depression or anxiety state.

- Organic psychosis requires less than acute functional psychosis, which in turn require less than chronic psychosis.

- An increased mortality rate in the post-operative period for psychotic patients receiving chronic antipsychotic therapy has been demonstrated.

Adverse responses during anesthesia

- Arrhythmias,
- Hypotension.
- Prolonged narcosis.
- Coma.
- Hyperpyrexia.
- Post-operative ileus.
- Post-operative confusion.
- Lack pain sensitivity and have pituitary–adrenal and autonomic nervous dysfunction.
- Abnormalities of the immune system.
- Water intoxication.
- These alterations may influence the post-operative outcome.

BIPOLAR DISORDERS
Valproate

- Lithium and valproate remain a mainstay of treatment. Lithium inhibits the release of thyroid hormones and results in hypothyroidism.

- Lithium is eliminated by the kidneys renal function is compromised
- There is dehydration, lithium levels rise dramatically.
- Toxic blood concentration produces confusion, sedation, muscle weakness tremors and slurred speech.
- Cardiac problems may include sinus bradycardia, sinus node dysfunction, AV block, T wave changes, hypotension and ventricular irritability.
- Lithium toxicity occurs when levels are >1.5 mmol/L, and is exacerbated by dehydration, diuretics and renal impairment.
- Lithium prolongs neuromuscular blockade and may decrease anaesthetic requirements because it blocks brainstem release of norepinephrine, epinephrine and dopamine.
- Drug interact.
- ions with lithium
- Thiazide diuretics reduce the clearance of lithium by the kidneys. Non-steroidal anti-inflammatory drugs may increase the lithium levels up to 40%, which can result in toxicity. Angiotensin converting enzyme inhibitors not only reduce the excretion of lithium but may also cause renal failure.
- Lithium prolongs neuromuscular blockade and may decrease anaesthetic requirements because it blocks brainstem release of norepinephrine, epinephrine and dopamine.
- The association of sedation with lithium suggests that anesthetic requirement may be decreased in these patients.

- Duration of both depolarizing and non-depolarizing muscle relaxants may be prolonged in the presence of lithium; therefore, neuromuscular monitoring should be used.

Neuroleptic or typical antipsychotics

- (chlorpromazine, haloperidol, trifluoperazine) cause extrapyramidal side-effects like acute dystonia, akathisia, Parkinsonism and tardive dyskinesia.
- Atypical antipsychotics (clozapine, olanzapine, risperidone, amisulpiride, quetiapine and aripiprazole), which do not have a tendency to cause extrapyramidal side-effects.
- They act via the D2 receptor blockade, but also act on other receptors like histamine (H1), serotonin (5HT2). acetylcholine (muscarinic) and alfa adrenergic receptors.
- Clozapine causes seizures and neutropenia. Weight gain, postural hypotension and gynaecomastia are also very common with antipsychotic drugs.

Anesthetics reaction with Neuroleptic or typical antipsychotics

- Effects of antipsychotic drugs include α-adrenergic blockade causing postural hypotension, prolongation of QT intervals, seizures, hepatic enzyme elevation, abnormal temperature regulation, sedation and Parkinsonism-like manifestations.
- Drug-induced sedation may decrease anesthetic requirement.

- The heart rate during anaesthesia tends to increase in schizophrenic patients due to the use of antipsychotic drugs

The risk factors for hypotension
- increased age,
- use of antihypertensives,
- Increased individual sensitivity to anesthetics and the influence of the renin–angiotensin system.
- Adjust the anesthetic dose according to individual response.
- Ketamine should probably be avoided as antipsychotics decrease the seizure threshold
- Increased body weight, diabetes mellitus and frequent smoking.
- Weight gain is a common problem in patients receiving antipsychotics.
- Antipsychotics can produce glucose intolerance by decreasing insulin action.
- Torsades de pointes and sudden death occurs in 10–15 of 10,000 patients taking antipsychotic drugs, which is almost twice as often as in normal populations.
- Paralytic ileus is caused by the anticholinergic and noradrenergic effect of antipsychotic drugs.
- Temperature regulation during anaesthesia may be impaired in chronic schizophrenic patients because of the direct effect on hypothalamic thermoregulation caused by dopamine blockade with antipsychotics

- hypersecretion of cortisols.
- Increased rate of infectious disease have been demonstrated in schizophrenic patients. This may be a consequence of dysregulation of the immune system.
- Life-threatening water intoxication often occurs in chronic schizophrenic patients.
- Water intoxication is associated with vasopressin hypersecretion as a result of chronic administration of antipsychotics.

NEUROLEPTIC MALIGNANT SYNDROME

- It causes acute hyperthermia,
- Muscular rigidity.
- Altered mental status.
- Elevated creatinine phosphokinase and autonomic dysfunction. Awareness of diagnosis, cessation of medication, early medical intervention and consideration of specific remedies can reduce morbidity and mortality when Neuroleptic Malignant Syndrome occurs.
- Patients should be treated in the intensive care unit. Dentrolene

References

1. Pumphrey CW, Fuster V, Chesebro JH; Systemic thromboembolism in valvular heart disease and prosthetic heart valves. Mod Concepts Cardiovasc Dis. 51 1982:131-136.

2. Fuster V, Gersh BJ, Giuliani ER; The natural history of idiopathic dilated cardiomyopathy. Am J Cardiol. 47 1981:525-531.

3. Wolf PA, Dawber TR, Thomas HE Jr; Epidemiologic assessment of chronic atrial fibrillation and risk of stroke: the Framingham Study. Neurology. 28 1978:973-977.

4. Coulshed N, Epstein EJ, McKendrick CS, Galloway RW, Walker E; Systemic embolism in mitral valve disease. Br Heart J. 32 1970:26-34.

5. Fleming HA, Bailey SM; Mitral valve disease, systemic embolism and anticoagulants. Postgrad Med J. 47 1971:599-604.

6. Szekely P; Systemic embolism and anticoagulant prophylaxis in rheumatic heart disease. Br Med J. 1 1964:1209-1212.

7. Easton JD, Sherman DG; Management of cerebral embolism of cardiac origin. Stroke. 11 1980:433-442.

8. Hart RG, Miller VT; Cerebral infarction in young adults: a practical approach. Stroke. 14 1983:110-114.

9. Deveral PB, Olley PM, Smith DR, Watson DA, Whitaker W; Incidence of systemic embolism before and after mitral valvotomy. Thorax. 23 1968:530-536.

10. Abernathy WS, Willis PW; Thromboembolic complications of rheumatic heart disease. Cardiovasc Clin. 5 1973:131-175.

11. Nielsen GH, Galea EG, Hossack KF; Thromboembolic complications of mitral valve disease. Aust NZ J Med. 8 1978:372-376.

12. Askey JM, Berstein S; The management of rheumatic heart disease in relation to systemic arterial embolism. Prog Cardiovasc Disease. 3 1960:220-232.

13. Fuster V, Pumphrey CW, McGoon MD, Chesebro JH. Systemic thromboembolism in mitral and aortic valve disease: a long-term follow up. Personal communication..

14. Nishimura RA, McGoon MD, Shub C, Miller FA, Ilstrup DM, Tajik AJ; Echocardiographically documented mitral-valve prolapse: longterm follow-up of 237 patients. N Engl J Med. 313 1985:1305-1309.

15. Savage DD, Garrison RJ, Devereaux RB; Mitral valve prolapse in the general population. I. Epidemiologic features: the Framingham Study. Am Heart 1. 106 1983:571-576.

16. Bamett HJ, Boughner DR, Taylor DW; Further evidence relating mitral-valve prolapse to cerebral ischemic events. N Engl J Med. 302 1980:139-144.

17. Barnett HIM, Jones MW, Boughner DR, Kostuk WJ; Cerebral ischemic events associated with prolapsing mitral valve. Arch Neurol. 33 1976:777-782.

18. Ritchie JL, Bateman TM, Bonow RO, et al. Guidelines for clinical use of cardiac radionuclide imaging: report of the American College of Cardiology/American Heart Association Task Force on Assessment of Diagnostic and Therapeutic Cardiovascular Procedures (Committee on Radionuclide Imaging), developed in collaboration with the American Society of Nuclear Cardiology. J Am Coll Cardiol. 1995;25:521–547.

19. Cheitlin MD, Alpert JS, Armstrong WF, et al. ACC/AHA guidelines for the clinical application of echocardiography: a report of the American College of Cardiology/American Heart Association Task Force on Practice Guidelines (Committee on Clinical Application of Echocardiography), developed in collaboration with the American Society of Echocardiography. Circulation.1997;95:1686–1744.

20. Gibbons RJ, Beasley JW, Bricker JT, et al. ACC/AHA guidelines for exercise testing: a report of the American College of Cardiology/American Heart Association Task Force on Practice Guidelines (Committee on Exercise Testing). J Am Coll Cardiol. 1997;30:260–311.

21. Scanlon PJ, Faxon DP, Audet AM, et al. ACC/AHA guidelines for coronary angiography: a report of the American College of Cardiology/American Heart Association Task Force on Practice Guidelines (Committee on Coronary Angiography). J Am Coll Cardiol. In press.

22. Dajani AS, Taubert KA, Wilson W, et al. Prevention of bacterial endocarditis: recommendations by the American Heart Association. Circulation.1997;96:358–366.

23. Dajani A, Taubert K, Ferrieri P, Peter G, Shulman S. Treatment of acute streptococcal pharyngitis and prevention of rheumatic fever: a statement for health professionals: Committee on Rheumatic Fever, Endocarditis, and Kawasaki Disease of the Council on Cardiovascular Disease in the Young, the American Heart Association. Pediatrics. 1995;96:758–764.

24. Cheitlin MD, Douglas PS, Parmley WW. 26th Bethesda conference: recommendations for determining eligibility for competition in athletes with cardiovascular abnormalities. Task Force 2: acquired valvular heart disease. J Am Coll Cardiol. 1994;24:874–880.

25. From the Centers for Disease Control and Prevention. Cardiac valvulopathy associated with exposure to fenfluramine and dexfenfluramine: US Department of Health and Human Services interim public health recommendations, November 1997. JAMA. 1997;278:1729–1731.

26. Curr Opin Anaesthesiol: 2002, 15(3);365-70

27. G Martucci, A Di Lorenzo, F Polito, L Acampa A 12-month follow-up for neurological complica Ihab R Dorotta, Armin Schubert Multiple sclerosis and anesthetic implications.tion after subarachnoid anesthesia in a parturient affected by multiple sclerosis. Eur Rev Med Pharmacol Sci: 2011, 15(4);458-60

28. Anaesthetic implications of anticancer chemotherapy.[Eur J Anaesthesiol. 2003]

29. Anaesthesia for cancer patients.[Curr Opin Anaesthesiol. 2007]

30. Anaesthetic issues in women undergoing gynaecological cytoreductive surgery.[Curr Opin Anaesthesiol. 2009]

31. Anaesthesia of farmed fish: implications for welfare.[Fish Physiol Biochem. 2012]

32. Anaesthesia for the patient with dementia undergoing outpatient surgery.[Curr Opin Anaesthesiol. 2009]

33. Huyse FJ, Touw DJ, Schijndel RS, Lange JJ, Slaets JP. Psychotropic drugs and the perioperative period: A proposal for a guideline in elective surgery. Psychosomatics. 2006;47:8–22. [PubMed]

34. Singh MK, Giles LL, Nasrallah HA. Pain insensitivity in schizophrenia: Trait or state marker? J PsychiatrPract.2006:90–102. [PubMed]

35. Kudoh A. Perioperative management of chronic schizophrenic patients. AnesthAnalg. 2005;101:1867–72.

36. Wik G. Effects of neuroleptic treatment on cortisol and 3-methoxy-4-hydroxyphenylethyl glycol levels in blood.J Endocrinol. 1995;144:425–9.

37. Naudin J, Capo C, Giusano B, Mege JL, Azorin JM. A differential role for interleukin-6 and tumor necrosis factor in schizophrenia? Schizophr Res. 1997;26:227–33.

38. Goldman MB, Robertson GL, Luchins DJ, Hedeker D, Pandey GN. Psychotic exacerbations and enhanced vasopressin secretion in schizophrenic patients with hyponatremia and polydipsia. Arch Gen Psychiatry.1997;54:443–9.

39. Morgan GE, Mikhail MS, Murray MJ. Morgan: Clinical anaesthesiology. 4th ed. USA: LANGE International edition; 2008. Anesthesia for patients with neurologic and psychiatric diseases; pp. 647–6

40. Howland RH. Potential adverse effects of discontinuing psychotropic drugs. J PsychosocNursMent Health Serv.2010;48:9–12.

41. Hines RL, Marschall KE. Psychiatric disease/substance abuse/drug overdose Stoelting's: Anaesthesia and co- existing diseases. 5th ed. Gurgaon (India): ELSEVIER A division of Reed Elsevier India Private Ltd; 2010.

42. Kudoh A, Katagai H, Takazawa T. Effect of preoperative discontinuation of antipsychotics in schizophrenic patients on outcome during and after anesthesia. Eur J Anaesth. 2004;21:414–6.

43. Sawada N, Higashi K, Yanagi F, Nishi M, Akasaka T, Kudoh J. Sudden onset of bronchospasm and persistent hypotension during spinal anesthesia in a patient on long-term psychotropic therapy. Masui.1997;46:1225–9.

44. 12. Lanctot KL, Best TS, Mittman N, Liu BA, Oh PI, Einarson TR, et al. Efficacy and safety of neuroleptics in behavioral disorders associated with dementia. J Clin Psychiatry. 1998;59:550–61.

45. Buckley NA, Sanders P. Cardiovascular adverse effects of antipsychotic drugs. Drug Saf. 2000;23:215–28.

46. Kudoh A, Kudo T, Ishihara H, Matsuki A. Depressed pituitary-adrenal response to surgical stress in chronic schizophrenic patients. Neuropsychobiol. 1997;36:112–6.

47. 15. Kawachi I. Physical and psychological consequence of weight gain. J Clin Psychiatry. 1999;60(Suppl 21):5–9.

48. Baptista T. Body weight gain induced by antipsychotic drugs: Mechanisms and management.ActaPsychiatrScand. 1999;100:3–16.

49. Glassman AH, Bigger JT., Jr Antipsychotic drugs: Prolonged QTc interval, torsade de pointes, and sudden death. Am J Psychiatry. 2001;158:1774–82.

50. Kudoh A, Ishihara H, Matsuki A. Pituitary-adrenal and parasympathetic function of chronic schizophrenic patients with postoperative ileus or hypotension. Neuropsychobiol. 1999;39:125–30. [

51. Patt RB, Proper G, Reddy S. The neuroleptics as adjuvant analgesics. J Pain Sympt Manage. 1994;9:446–53.

52. Young DM. Risk factors for hypothermia in psychiatric patients. Ann Clin Psychiatry. 1996;8:93–7.

53. Molnar G, Fava GA. Principles of medical psychiatry. Orland: Gruneand Stratton Inc; 1987. Intercurrent medical illness in the schizophrenic patients; p. 451.

54. O'Keeffe ST, Devlin JG. Delirium and the dexamethasone suppression test in the elderly. Neuropsychobiol.1994;30:153–6.

55. Van der Mast RC. Pathophysiology of delirium. J Geriatr Psychiatry Neurol. 1998;11:138–45.

56. Agrawal P, Agrawal A, Singh I. Neuroleptic malignant syndrome and anaesthesia: A case report. The Indian Anaesthetists Forum. 2010. Jan, [Last cited on 2011 July 10].

57. Klotz U. Tramadol-the impact of its pharmacokinetic and pharmacodynamic properties on the clinical management of pain. Arzneimittelforschung. 2003;53:681–7.

www.ingramcontent.com/pod-product-compliance
Lightning Source LLC
Chambersburg PA
CBHW070228210526
45169CB00023B/1258